I0483737

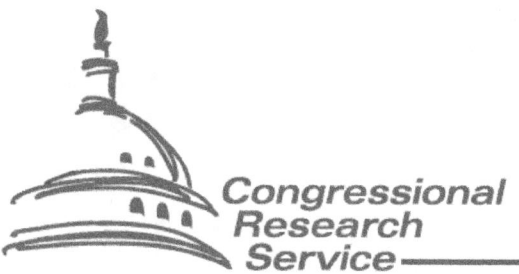

Congressional Research Service

Medicaid Financing and Expenditures

Alison Mitchell
Analyst in Health Care Financing

July 30, 2012

Congressional Research Service

7-5700

www.crs.gov

R42640

CRS Report for Congress

Prepared for Members and Committees of Congress

Summary

Medicaid is a means-tested entitlement program that finances the delivery of primary and acute medical services as well as long-term services and supports. Medicaid is a federal and state partnership that is jointly financed by both the federal government and the states.

The federal government's share for most Medicaid expenditures is called the federal medical assistance percentage (FMAP) rate. Generally determined annually, the FMAP formula is designed so that the federal government pays a larger portion of Medicaid costs in states with lower per capita incomes relative to the national average (and vice versa for states with higher per capita incomes). Federal Medicaid funding to states is open-ended.

The federal government provides states a good deal of flexibility in determining the composition of the state share (also referred to as the non-federal share) of Medicaid expenditures. As a result, there is significant variation from state to state in the funding sources used to finance the state share of Medicaid expenditures. In state fiscal year 2010, states reported that on average state general funds (i.e., revenues from personal income, sales, and corporate income taxes) made up 76% of the state share of Medicaid expenditures and the remaining 24% was financed by "other state funds" (i.e., provider taxes, local government funds, and tobacco settlement funds).

In FY2011, Medicaid expenditures totaled $428 billion, with the federal government paying $271 billion, about 63% of the total. While Medicaid expenditures (like all health expenditures) generally grow at a rate faster than the economy, as measured by the gross domestic product (GDP), spending per enrollee under Medicaid tends to be lower than the per person spending for other forms of health insurance. One of the major factors impacting Medicaid spending is the economy. Also, state-specific factors, such as programmatic decisions and demographics, affect Medicaid expenditures and cause Medicaid spending to vary widely from state to state.

Starting in FY2014, Medicaid expenditures are expected to increase significantly as a result of the reforms enacted in the Patient Protection and Affordable Care Act (ACA, P.L. 111-148 as amended). The most noteworthy ACA change to Medicaid begins in 2014, or sooner at state option, when some states expand Medicaid eligibility to adults under age 65 with income up to 133% of the federal poverty level (FPL) (effectively 138% FPL with the Modified Adjusted Gross Income 5% FPL income disregard).

Following the June 28, 2012, Supreme Court decision in *National Federation of Independent Business v. Sebelius*, it is uncertain how many states will refuse to expand their Medicaid program to cover this new group. The Congressional Budget Office and the Joint Committee on Taxation updated their estimate of the ACA Medicaid expansion to account for the Supreme Court decision, and they project the expansion will cost $642 billion from FY2014 to FY2022, which is $288 billion less than the estimate prior to the Supreme Court decision.

This report provides an overview of Medicaid's financing structure, including both federal and state financing issues. The Medicaid expenditures section of the report discusses economic factors affecting Medicaid, state variability in spending, and projected program spending. Other issues that are examined include congressional proposals to turn Medicaid into a block grant program, federal deficit reduction proposals affecting Medicaid, and state fiscal conditions affecting Medicaid financing and services.

Contents

Figures

Contacts

Introduction

Medicaid is a means-tested entitlement[1] program that finances the delivery of primary and acute medical services as well as long-term services and supports.[2] Medicaid is a federal and state partnership. The states are responsible for administering their Medicaid programs, and Medicaid is jointly financed by the federal government and the states. In FY2011, Medicaid is estimated to have provided health care services to 56 million individuals[3] at a total cost of $428 billion (including federal and state expenditures).[4]

Participation in Medicaid is voluntary, though all states, the District of Columbia, and the territories choose to participate. The federal government sets some basic requirements[5] for Medicaid, but states are provided flexibility to design their own version of Medicaid within the federal government's basic framework.

States incur Medicaid costs by making payments to service providers (e.g., for beneficiaries' doctor visits) and performing administrative activities (e.g., making eligibility determinations). The federal government reimburses states for a share of each dollar spent in accordance with their federally approved Medicaid state plans.

Medicaid is an entitlement for both states and individuals. The Medicaid entitlement to states ensures that, so long as states operate their programs within the federal requirements, states are entitled to federal Medicaid matching funds. This means that federal Medicaid spending is open-ended. Medicaid is also an individual entitlement, which means that anyone eligible for Medicaid under his or her state's eligibility standards is guaranteed Medicaid coverage.

This report provides an overview of Medicaid's financing structure including both federal and state financing issues. The Medicaid expenditures section of the report discusses economic factors affecting Medicaid, state variability in spending, and projected program spending. Other issues that are examined include congressional proposals to turn Medicaid into a block grant program, federal deficit reduction proposals affecting Medicaid, and state fiscal conditions affecting Medicaid financing and services.

---

[1] Entitlement means that individuals who meet state eligibility requirements, which must also meet federal minimum requirements, are entitled to Medicaid coverage.

[2] For more information about the Medicaid program, see CRS Report RL33202, *Medicaid A Primer*, by Elicia J. Herz.

[3] This enrollment figure is measured according to "person-year equivalents," which is the average enrollment over the course of a year. Christopher J. Truffer, John D. Klemm, and Christian J. Wolfe, et al., *2011 Actuarial Report on the Financial Outlook for Medicaid*, Centers for Medicare & Medicaid Services' Office of the Actuary, March 2012.

[4] U.S. Department of Health and Human Services, Centers for Medicare and Medicaid Services, Form CMS-64 data, April 2012.

[5] The federal government requires states cover certain populations and benefits. On June 28, 2012, the United States Supreme Court issued its decision in *National Federation of Independent Business v. Sebelius*, finding that the federal government cannot terminate current Medicaid program federal matching funds if a state refuses to implement the Medicaid expansion required by the Patient Protection and Affordable Care Act (ACA, P.L. 111-148), which expands Medicaid eligibility to include non-elderly, non-pregnant adults under 133% of the federal poverty level. If a state accepts the new ACA Medicaid expansion funds, it must abide by the new expansion coverage rules, but, based on the Court's opinion, it appears that a state can refuse to participate in the expansion without losing any of its current federal Medicaid matching funds.

Medicaid Financing

The federal government and the states share the cost of Medicaid. The federal government reimburses states for a portion (i.e., the federal share) of each state's Medicaid program costs. Because federal Medicaid funding is an open-ended entitlement to states, there is no upper limit or cap on the amount of federal Medicaid funds a state may receive. In a typical year, the federal share of Medicaid expenditures is about 57%, which means the state share is about 43%.[6]

Federal Share

A primary goal of the federal Medicaid matching arrangement is to share the cost of providing health care services to low-income residents with the states. The Medicaid financing structure represents a clear fiscal commitment on the part of the federal government toward paying at least half (but not all) of the cost of Medicaid.[7]

The federal government's open-ended financial commitment to Medicaid provides a fiscal incentive for states to extend Medicaid coverage to more low-income individuals than a state might choose to fund without the federal Medicaid funding. However, this incentive is counterbalanced by the requirement for states to share in the cost of Medicaid.[8,9]

The Federal Medical Assistance Percentage (FMAP) Rate

The federal government's share of most Medicaid expenditures is established by the FMAP rate, which is generally determined annually and varies by state according to each state's per capita income relative to the U.S. per capita income.[10] The formula provides higher FMAP rates, or federal reimbursement rates, to states with lower per capita incomes and lower FMAP rates to states with higher per capita incomes. FMAP rates have a statutory minimum of 50% and a statutory maximum of 83%.[11] The formula for a given state is

$$\text{FMAP}_{state} = 1 - ((\text{Per capita income}_{state})^2/(\text{Per capita income}_{U.S.})^2 * 0.45)$$

---

[6] For FY2009 through FY2011, the federal share of Medicaid expenditures was higher than usual due to the temporary FMAP increase provided to states from October 1, 2008 through June 30, 2011. The temporary FMAP increase was originally provided through the American Recovery and Reinvestment Act of 2009 (P.L. 111-5) and extended through P.L. 111-226. For more information about the temporary FMAP increase, see CRS Report RL32950, *Medicaid The Federal Medical Assistance Percentage (FMAP)*, by Alison Mitchell and Evelyne P. Baumrucker.

[7] Andy Schneider and David Rousseau, *The Medicaid Resource Book*, The Kaiser Commission on Medicaid and the Uninsured, Publication Number 2236, January 17, 2003; Teresa A. Coughlin and Stephen Zuckerman, *States' Use of Medicaid Maximization Strategies to Tap Federal Revenues Program Implications and Consequences*, The Urban Institute, June 2002.

[8] Ibid.

[9] State decisions regarding Medicaid eligibility levels are determined based on a number of state-specific factors, including policy decisions about which optional eligibility groups should receive Medicaid coverage.

[10] For more detail about FMAP, see CRS Report RL32950, *Medicaid The Federal Medical Assistance Percentage (FMAP)*, by Alison Mitchell and Evelyne P. Baumrucker.

[11] Section 1905(b) of the Social Security Act.

The use of the 0.45 factor in the formula is designed to ensure that a state with per capita income equal to the U.S. average receives an FMAP rate of 55%, with a state share of 45%. In addition, the formula's squaring of per capita income provides higher FMAP rates to states with below-average per capita incomes than the states would otherwise receive (and vice versa).[12] In FY2012, FMAP rates range from 50% (14 states) to 74% (Mississippi).

Exceptions to the FMAP Rate and Open-Ended Funding

The FMAP rate is used to reimburse states for the federal share of most Medicaid expenditures, but exceptions to the regular FMAP rate have been made for certain states (e.g., the District of Columbia and the territories), situations (e.g., during economic downturns), populations (e.g., certain women with breast or cervical cancer and individuals in the Qualifying Individuals[13] program), providers (e.g., primary care physicians and Indian Health Service facilities), and services (e.g., family planning and home health services).[14] In addition, the federal share for most Medicaid administrative costs does not vary by state and is generally 50%.

While most federal Medicaid funding is provided on an open-ended basis, certain types of federal Medicaid funding are capped. For instance, federal disproportionate share hospital (DSH)[15] funding to states cannot exceed a state-specific annual allotment. Also, Medicaid programs in the territories (i.e., American Samoa, Guam, Northern Mariana Islands, Puerto Rico, and the Virgin Islands) are subject to annual spending caps. Other exceptions to open-ended federal Medicaid funding include the Qualified Individuals program and waivers that allow states to operate outside of normal federal rules (which are subject to aggregate budget caps or cost-per-beneficiary caps).[16]

Medicaid and the Federal Budget Process

As discussed above, Medicaid is a federal entitlement to states, and in federal budget parlance entitlement spending is categorized as mandatory spending, which is also referred to as direct spending. However, Medicaid is an unusual mandatory spending program.

While most mandatory spending programs bypass the annual appropriations process and automatically receive funding each year according to either permanent or multi-year

---

[12] For example, assume that U.S. per capita income is $40,000. In state A with a *below-average* per capita income of $38,000, the FMAP formula produces an FMAP rate of 59.39%; if the formula did not include a squaring of per capita income, it would instead produce a lower FMAP rate of 57.25%. In state B with an *above-average* per capita income of $42,000, the FMAP formula produces an FMAP rate of 50.39%; if the formula did not include a squaring of per capita income, it would instead produce a higher FMAP rate of 52.75%.

[13] States are required to pay Medicare Part B premiums for Medicare beneficiaries with income between 120% and 135% FPL and limited assets (referred to as "qualifying individuals"), up to a specified dollar allotment.

[14] For more detail about the FMAP exceptions, see CRS Report RL32950, *Medicaid The Federal Medical Assistance Percentage (FMAP)*, by Alison Mitchell and Evelyne P. Baumrucker.

[15] The federal Medicaid statute requires that states make disproportionate share (DSH) adjustments to the payment rates of hospitals treating large numbers of low-income and Medicaid patients.

[16] In addition, some states have chosen to expand their Medicaid programs using capped federal allotments for the State Children's Health Insurance Program (CHIP). However, this does not affect the open-ended nature of federal funding for Medicaid. Once these states have exhausted their CHIP allotments, they revert to using Medicaid funds. For more information about CHIP, see CRS Report R40444, *State Children's Health Insurance Program (CHIP) A Brief Overview*, by Elicia J. Herz and Evelyne P. Baumrucker.

---

appropriations in the substantive law, Medicaid is funded in the annual appropriations acts. For this reason, Medicaid is referred to as an "appropriated entitlement."[17]

The level of spending for appropriated entitlements, like other entitlements, is based on the benefit and eligibility criteria established in law. The amount of budget authority provided in appropriations acts for Medicaid is based on budget projections for meeting the funding needs of the program. While most changes to the Medicaid program are made through statute, the fact that Medicaid is subject to annual appropriations process provides an opportunity for Congress to place funding limitations on specified activities in Medicaid, including the circumstances under which federal funds can be used to pay for abortions.

State Share

The federal government provides broad guidelines to states regarding allowable funding sources for the state share (also referred to as the non-federal share) of Medicaid expenditures. However, to a large extent, states are free to determine how to fund their share of Medicaid expenditures. As a result, there is significant variation from state to state in funding sources.

States can use state general funds (i.e., personal income, sales, and corporate income taxes) and "other state funds" (i.e., provider taxes, local government funds, tobacco settlement funds, etc.) to finance the state share of Medicaid.[18] Federal statute[19] allows as much as 60% of the state share to come from local government funding.[20] Federal regulations also stipulate that the state share not be funded with federal funds (Medicaid or otherwise).[21] In state fiscal year (SFY) 2010, on average, 76% of the state share of Medicaid expenditures was financed by state general funds, and the remaining 24% was financed by "other state funds." [22]

A few funding sources have received a great deal of attention over the past couple decades because states have used these funds in some financing mechanisms designed to maximize the amount of federal Medicaid funds coming to the state. This is referred to as "Medicaid maximization."[23] In general, some states have used "Medicaid maximization" strategies that

---

[17] For more information about "appropriated entitlements," see CRS Report RS20129, *Entitlements and Appropriated Entitlements in the Federal Budget Process*, by Bill Heniff Jr.

[18] Ibid.

[19] Section 1902(a)(2) of the Social Security Act.

[20] The federal statute allows for the significant use of local funds in financing Medicaid because local governments financed a significant amount of the health care services provided to low-income individuals prior to the enactment of Medicaid. The Patient Protection and Affordable Care Act (ACA, P.L. 111-148) included a provision that restricts states from increasing required local contributions to the state share of Medicaid. Specifically, in the case of a state that requires a political subdivision within the state to contribute to the non-federal share of expenditures, such state would not be eligible for an increase in its FMAP rate (under ACA or the American Recovery and Reinvestment Act of 2009, P.L. 111-5) if the state requires that political subdivisions pay a greater percentage of the non-federal share of expenditures (including expenditures for DSH payments) than amounts that would have been required as of December 31, 2009. Voluntary contributions are not considered "required" contributions. (Medicaid and CHIP Payment and Access Commission, *Report to the Congress on Medicaid and CHIP*, March 2012.)

[21] 42 C.F.R. 433.51(c).

[22] National Association of State Budget Officers, *Fiscal Year 2010 State Expenditure Report Examining Fiscal 2009-2011 State Spending*, December 2011.

[23] National Health Policy Forum at The George Washington University, *The Basics Medicaid Financing*, February 4, 2011; U.S. Government Accountability Office, *Medicaid Financing Long-Standing Concerns about Inappropriate State Arrangements Support Need for Improved Federal Oversight*, testimony of Marjorie Kanof before U.S. Congress, (continued...)

---

involve the coordination of fund sources, such as provider taxes and intergovernmental transfers (IGTs), and payment policies, such as DSH and supplemental payments[24] to draw down federal Medicaid funds without expending much, if any, state general funds.

Provider Taxes

States are able to use revenues from health care provider taxes to help finance their share of Medicaid expenditures.[25] Federal statute and regulations define a provider tax as a health care-related fee, assessment, or other mandatory payment for which at least 85% of the burden of the tax revenue falls on health care providers.[26]

In order for states to be able to use the revenue generated from a provider tax to fund their state share of Medicaid expenditures, the provider tax must be both broad-based (i.e., imposed on all providers within a specified class of providers) and uniform (i.e., the same tax for all providers within a specified class of providers). Also, states are not allowed to hold the providers harmless for the cost of the provider tax (i.e., they cannot guarantee that providers receive their money back). In addition, provider tax revenue is prohibited from exceeding 25% of the state share of Medicaid expenditures.

States first began using health care provider taxes, as well as provider donations,[27] to help finance the state share of Medicaid expenditures in the mid-1980s. In some cases, Medicaid providers initiated these provider tax and donation arrangements because states would often use the resulting revenue to increase Medicaid payment rates. Plus, these arrangements were often designed in such a way as to hold the Medicaid providers harmless for the cost of their taxes or donations (i.e., providers received their tax and donation money back through Medicaid rate increases).[28]

While not all states were using provider taxes to finance their share of Medicaid, some states were particularly aggressive in their use of provider taxes. As a result, in 1991, Congress passed the Medicaid Voluntary Contribution and Provider-Specific Tax Amendments (P.L. 102-234) to

---

(...continued)

House of Representatives, Committee on Oversight and Government Reform, GAO-08-255T, November 1, 2007; Andy Schneider and David Rousseau, *The Medicaid Resource Book*, The Kaiser Commission on Medicaid and the Uninsured, Publication Number 2236, January 17, 2003; Teresa A. Coughlin and Stephen Zuckerman, *States' Use of Medicaid Maximization Strategies to Tap Federal Revenues Program Implications and Consequences*, The Urban Institute, June 2002.

[24] Supplemental payments are Medicaid payments made to providers that are separate from and in addition to the standard payment rates for services rendered to Medicaid enrollees. Often, providers receive supplemental payments in a lump sum.

[25] For more information about Medicaid provider taxes, see CRS Report RS22843, *Medicaid Provider Taxes*, by Alison Mitchell.

[26] The statute regarding provider taxes can be found in Section 1903(w) of the Social Security Act, and the accompanying regulations can be found at 42 C.F.R. 433.

[27] Provider donations are any donation or other voluntary payment made to a state or unit of local government by a health care provider. Section 1903(w)(2) of the Social Security Act.

[28] Andy Schneider, Risa Elias, Rachel Garfield, David Rousseau, and Victoria Wachino, *The Medicaid Resource Book*, Kaiser Commission on Medicaid and the Uninsured, July 2002.

---

restrict the use of provider donations in financing Medicaid to extremely limited situations[29] and to limit states' ability to use provider tax revenue to qualify for federal Medicaid matching funds.

A number of states[30] have approved additional provider taxes since the beginning of the most recent recession (December 2007 through June 2009),[31] despite federal statutory and regulatory limitations.[32] In SFY2012, 47 states and the District of Columbia used at least one provider tax to finance Medicaid.[33]

Provider taxes continue to cause tension between the federal government and the states. For this reason, some federal deficit reduction proposals recommend limiting states' ability to use provider taxes for Medicaid.[34]

Local Government Funds

As long as total local funds comprise less than 60% of the state share of Medicaid expenditures, local governments and local government providers can contribute to the state share of Medicaid payments through IGTs or certified public expenditures (CPEs). For IGTs, a local government transfers funds to the state government to be used to finance Medicaid. When CPEs are used to fund the state share, the local government certifies its Medicaid expenditures to the state, and then the state claims the federal Medicaid matching funds.[35]

Intergovernmental Transfers (IGTs)

IGTs are transfers of public funds between government entities, such as from counties to states or between state agencies. This financing mechanism is commonly used to enable states and local governments to carry out shared functions.

---

[29] Provider donations are permissible if they do not exceed $5,000 per year in the case of an individual provider or $50,000 per year in the case of a "health care organization entity" (42 C.F.R. 433.66(a)(1)). Also, provider donations are allowed if the donations are made by a hospital, clinic, or similar entity (such as federally qualified health centers) for the direct costs of state or local agency personnel who are stationed at the facility to determine the eligibility of individuals for Medicaid or to provide outreach services to eligible (or potentially eligible) Medicaid individuals (i.e., outstationed eligibility workers) (42 C.F.R. 433.66(a)(2)). Provider donations for outstationed eligibility workers may not exceed 10% of a state's administrative costs for the Medicaid program (42 C.F.R. 433.67).

[30] Action to generate additional provider tax revenue was taken by 4 states in SFY2009, 17 states in SFY2010, 10 states in SFY2011, and 12 states in SFY2012.

[31] Recession dates are designated by the National Bureau of Economic Research (NBER).

[32] The National Governors Association and the National Association of State Budget Officers, *The Fiscal Survey of States,* various years.

[33] Vernon K. Smith, Kathleen Gifford, Eileen Ellis et al., *Moving Ahead Amid Fiscal Challenges A Look at Medicaid Spending, Coverage and Policy Trends, Results from a 50-State Medicaid Budget Survey for State Fiscal Years 2011 and 2012,* Kaiser Commission on Medicaid and the Uninsured, October 2011.

[34] Department of Health and Human Services, *Fiscal Year 2013 Budget in Brief Strengthening Health and Opportunity for All Americans,* February 2012; The National Commission on Fiscal Responsibility and Reform, *The Moment of Truth,* December 2010; Congressional Budget Office, *Budget Options Volume I Health Care,* December 2008.

[35] U.S. Government Accountability Office, *Medicaid CMS Needs More Information on the Billions of Dollars Spent on Supplemental Payments,* GAO-08-614, May 2008.

The federal government allows the use of IGTs in financing the state share of Medicaid expenditures.[36] In fact, some states require their counties to transfer certain local tax revenues to help fund the state share of Medicaid expenditures for certain government providers (e.g., community mental health centers or hospitals) located in these counties.[37] For example, New York requires counties to pay roughly 30% of the state share of Medicaid, which is 15% of total Medicaid expenditures for New York.[38]

IGTs are a legitimate state budget tool, but IGTs become problematic when they are used in financing schemes that draw down excess federal Medicaid matching funds without using much, if any, state general funds.[39] Specifically, some states use IGTs to fund supplemental payments in order to leverage federal Medicaid matching funds.

An example of this would be if a state Medicaid program made a $20 million supplemental payment to a local health care facility and then requested the federal Medicaid matching funds for the supplemental payment. With an FMAP rate of 50%, both the federal government and the state would fund $10 million of the supplemental payment. The point at which this type of financing mechanism becomes contentious is when some states have the local health care facility transfer back to the state most of the supplemental payment (e.g., $18 million of the $20 million payment) through an IGT. In this example, the local health care facility retains $2 million, the state nets $8 million to use for other Medicaid or non-Medicaid purposes, and the federal government paid $10 million.[40]

Certified Public Expenditures (CPEs)

CPEs are another way for states to use local government funds to finance the state share of Medicaid. Under a CPE, either state or local governmental entities, including government-owned providers (e.g., county hospitals or local education agencies) make Medicaid expenditures according to the state's approved Medicaid state plan. Then, the government entity certifies to the state Medicaid agency that the expenditures are eligible for federal Medicaid matching funds. Once the state receives this certification, the state can draw down the federal matching funds.

---

[36] Section 1903(w)(6) of the Social Security Act. 42 CFR 433.51.

[37] U.S. Government Accountability Office, *Medicaid CMS Needs More Information on the Billions of Dollars Spent on Supplemental Payments*, GAO-08-614, May 2008.; National Health Policy Forum at The George Washington University, *The Basics Medicaid Financing*, February 4, 2011; Medicaid and CHIP Payment and Access Commission, *Report to the Congress on Medicaid and CHIP*, March 2012.

[38] Michael Birnbaum, *Medicaid in New York Current Roles, Recent Experience, and Implications of Federal Reform*, Medicaid Institute at United Hospital Fund, December 2010.

[39] U.S. General Accounting Office, *Medicaid Intergovernmental Transfers Have Facilitated State Financing Schemes*, GAO-04-574T, March 18, 2004; National Health Policy Forum at The George Washington University, *The Basics Medicaid Financing*, February 4, 2011; Teresa A. Coughlin and Stephen Zuckerman, *States' Use of Medicaid Maximization Strategies to Tap Federal Revenues Program Implications and Consequences*, The Urban Institute, June 2002.

[40] U.S. Government Accountability Office, *Medicaid Financing Federal Oversight Initiative Is Consistent with Medicaid Payment Principles but Needs Greater Oversight*, GAO-07-214, March 2007.; U.S. General Accounting Office, *Medicaid Intergovernmental Transfers Have Facilitated State Financing Schemes*, GAO-04-574T, March 18, 2004; Teresa A. Coughlin and Stephen Zuckerman, *States' Use of Medicaid Maximization Strategies to Tap Federal Revenues Program Implications and Consequences*, The Urban Institute, June 2002.

Federal statute[41] specifies that the funds used to finance Medicaid through a CPE must be derived from state or local taxes.[42]

States employ CPEs differently. Some states use CPEs with local health department, and other states use CPEs with hospitals operated by state/local governments. CPEs are also commonly used for Medicaid services provided at schools. Specifically, local education agencies certify Medicaid expenditures for Medicaid school-based health care and related administrative services. Then, the state draws down the federal matching funds.[43]

Process for Federal Medicaid Funds Getting to States

States incur Medicaid costs by making payments to service providers (e.g., for beneficiaries' doctor visits) and performing administrative activities (e.g., making eligibility determinations). After a state has made Medicaid expenditures, it can draw down federal matching funds. The Medicaid financing structure is set up so that states can draw down federal Medicaid matching funds on a real time basis, and the federal government reconciles state Medicaid expenditures on a quarterly basis.[44]

The Centers for Medicare & Medicaid Services (CMS) makes quarterly grant awards to states to cover the federal share of Medicaid expenditures. The amount of each quarterly grant is determined on the basis of quarterly estimates submitted to CMS by each state's Medicaid agency on the Form CMS-37 at least 45 days before the beginning of each fiscal quarter.

After CMS analyzes states' estimates, states receive grant awards that authorize them to draw down federal funds as needed to pay the federal share of Medicaid expenditures. States draw down federal matching funds through commercial banks and the Federal Reserve System against a continuing letter of credit certified by the Secretary of the Treasury in favor of the state payee.[45]

Each state must submit a Form CMS-64 no later than 30 days after the end of each quarter with the state's accounting of actual recorded expenditures. CMS reviews the expenditures reported on the CMS-64 to reconcile the states' estimates from the CMS-37 with the actual documented expenditures to ensure that the reported expenditures are allowable under the Medicaid statute.

In order to qualify for federal Medicaid matching funds, state Medicaid expenditures must be allowable. If CMS is uncertain as to whether a particular state expenditure is allowable, then CMS must notify the state and provide an opportunity for a hearing. If the state does not comply, CMS may withhold payment or disallow claims for federal Medicaid matching funds until the issue has been resolved.[46]

---

[41] Section 1903(w)(6) of the Social Security Act. 42 CFR 433.51.

[42] Medicaid and CHIP Payment and Access Commission , *Report to the Congress on Medicaid and CHIP*, March 2012.

[43] Ibid.

[44] 42 C.F.R. 430.30.

[45] Ibid.

[46] 42 C.F.R. 430.35 and 42 C.F.R. 430.42

Medicaid Expenditures[47]

Medicaid expenditures account for a significant portion of total health expenditures in the United States. While Medicaid expenditures (like all health expenditures) generally grow at a rate faster than the economy as measured by the gross domestic product (GDP), spending per enrollee under Medicaid tends to be lower than the per-enrollee spending for other forms of health insurance. One of the major factors impacting Medicaid spending is the economy. Also, state-specific factors, such as policy decisions and demographics, impact Medicaid expenditures and cause Medicaid spending to vary widely from state to state. Estimating the growth of Medicaid expenditures is uncertain due to the Supreme Court decision in *National Federation of Independent Business v. Sebelius*.

Medicaid in Terms of National Health Expenditures

In calendar year 2010, Medicaid expenditures were 15.5% of all health expenditures in the United States, including acute care services, long-term services and supports, and administrative expenditures. Medicaid pays for a significant portion of all long-term services and supports. In 2010, Medicaid paid for 31.5% of all nursing facility and continuing care retirement community expenditures, 37.3% of all home health care expenditures, and 52.7% of all other health, residential, and personal care expenditures. Medicaid's share of national health expenditures for other services is relatively smaller, with Medicaid expenditures accounting for 18.7% of all hospital expenditures, 8.3% of all physician and clinical expenditures, and 7.1% of all dental expenditures.[48]

Trend in Medicaid Expenditures

From the program's inception in 1966, the cost of Medicaid, like most health expenditures, has generally increased at a rate significantly faster than the economy as measured by GDP. In the past, much of Medicaid's expenditure growth has been due to federal or state expansions of Medicaid eligibility criteria,[49] but the per-enrollee costs for Medicaid have also increased faster than the economy as measured by GDP. However, when compared to other forms of health insurance, Medicaid per-enrollee expenditures are relatively low.[50]

Figure 1 shows Medicaid expenditures from FY1997 to FY2011. These expenditures are broken down by the state expenditures, federal expenditures, and recession-related additional federal funding.

---

[47] Data in this section are provided for different years (i.e., FY2011, FY2010, or calendar year 2010) because Medicaid data are collected from states at different times for different purposes. For each type of expenditure, the most recent data are provided.

[48] Centers for Medicare & Medicaid Services, National Health Expenditures Data, 2010.

[49] Rachel Garfield, Lisa Clemans-Cope, and Emily Lawton, et al., *Enrollment-Driven Expenditure Growth Medicaid Spending during the Economic Downturn, FFY2007-2010*, Kaiser Commission on Medicaid and the Uninsured, Publication #8309, May 2012.

[50] Christopher J. Truffer, John D. Klemm, and Christian J. Wolfe, et al., *2011 Actuarial Report on the Financial Outlook for Medicaid*, Centers for Medicare & Medicaid Services' Office of the Actuary, March 2012.

Figure 1. Federal and State Medicaid Expenditures
FY1997 to FY2011

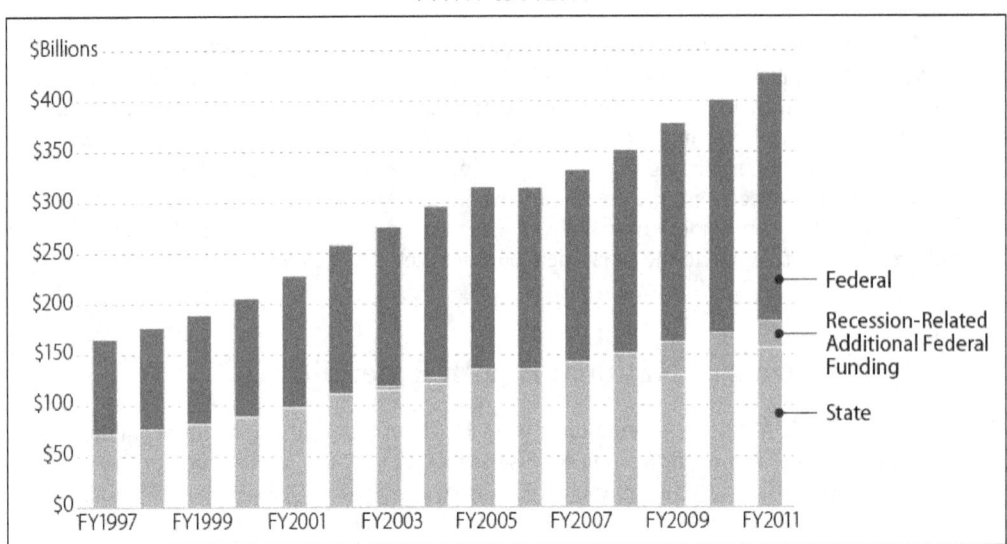

Source: Centers for Medicare & Medicaid, Form CMS-64 Data (the FY2011 CMS-64 data is pre iminary as of April 16, 2012), and Congressional Research Service communication with CMS from June 2012.

Note: Recession-related additional federal Medicaid funding was provided in response to the 2001 recession and the 2007-2009 recession. For the 2001 recession, additional federal funding was provided through the Job Growth and Tax Re ief Reconciliation Act of 2003 (P.L. 108-27). For the most recent recession, additional federal funding was provided through the American Recovery and Reinvestment Act of 2009 (ARRA, P.L. 111-5) and P.L. 111-226.

In FY2011, Medicaid spending on services and administrative activities in the 50 states, the District of Columbia, and the territories totaled $428 billion. Federal Medicaid expenditures totaled $271 billion with the regular federal share equaling $245 billion and additional, recession-related federal funds at $26 billion.[51] State Medicaid expenditures were $157 billion in FY2011, which was 37% of total Medicaid spending.[52]

---

[51] Additional federal Medicaid funding was provided in response to the 2001 recession through the Job Growth and Tax Relief Reconciliation Act of 2003 (P.L. 108-27), which provided temporary relief to states through a combination of grants and an increase in the FMAP for FY2003 and FY2004. For the most recent recession, fiscal relief was provided to states through the American Recovery and Reinvestment Act of 2009 (ARRA, P.L. 111-5), which provided states with a temporary FMAP rate increase and a reduction to the required payments for Medicare Part D (i.e., the "clawback" provision). The temporary FMAP increase was originally provided through ARRA for nine fiscal quarters (October 1, 2008 through December 31, 2010), and the temporary FMAP increase was extended by six months (January 1, 2011 through June 30, 2011) at a phased down level through P.L. 111-226. For more information about these temporary FMAP increases, see CRS Report RL32950, *Medicaid The Federal Medical Assistance Percentage (FMAP)*, by Alison Mitchell and Evelyne P. Baumrucker.

[52] U.S. Department of Health and Human Services, Centers for Medicare and Medicaid Services, Form CMS-64 data, April 16, 2012. The FY2011 CMS-64 data is preliminary.

Per-Enrollee Medicaid Expenditures

Per-enrollee Medicaid expenditures averaged $6,775 in FY2010.[53] However, as shown in **Figure 2**, per-enrollee expenditures varied significantly by population group (i.e., children, adults, aged, and disabled) with the per-enrollee expenditures by population group ranging from $2,717 for children to $16,963 for disabled individuals.

Figure 2. Expenditures Per Medicaid Enrollee by Major Population Groups

FY2010

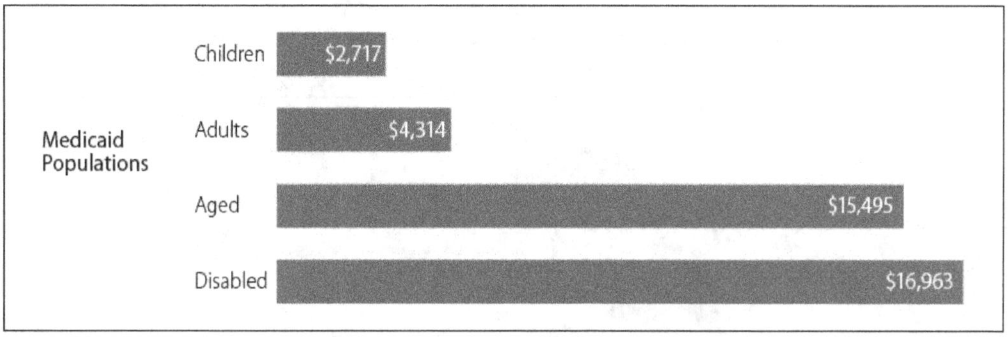

Source: Christopher J. Truffer, John D. Klemm, and Christian J. Wolfe, et al., *2011 Actuarial Report on the Financial Outlook for Medicaid*, Centers for Medicare & Medicaid Services' Office of the Actuary, March 2012.

Notes: Enrollment is measured in person-year equivalents, which is the average enrollment over the course of the year. This chart does not include expenditures for DSH, the territories, or adjustments (i.e., net adjustments of benefits from prior periods and the difference between expenditures and outlays).

One reason the aged and disabled populations have higher per-enrollee expenditures is because these populations consume most of the long-term services and supports, which comprise almost a quarter of all Medicaid expenditures (see **Figure 3**). Another reason for the difference in per-enrollee expenditures by population group is that children and adults tend to be healthier and therefore tend to have lower health care costs than the aged and disabled populations, even though a significant number of non-disabled adults are pregnant women.[54]

In FY2010, the aged and disabled populations together accounted for about 27% of Medicaid enrollment and 66% of Medicaid expenditures. In comparison, the children and adult populations accounted for about 74% of Medicaid enrollment and 34% of Medicaid expenditures.[55]

---

[53] This figure excludes Medicaid expenditures for DSH, the territories, and administrative costs. Also, this figure is based on Medicaid enrollment measured by person-year equivalents, which is the average enrollment over the course of a year. Christopher J. Truffer, John D. Klemm, and Christian J. Wolfe, et al., *2011 Actuarial Report on the Financial Outlook for Medicaid*, Centers for Medicare & Medicaid Services' Office of the Actuary, March 2012.

[54] Andy Schneider and David Rousseau, *The Medicaid Resource Book*, The Kaiser Commission on Medicaid and the Uninsured, Publication Number 2236, January 17, 2003.

[55] Christopher J. Truffer, John D. Klemm, and Christian J. Wolfe, et al., *2011 Actuarial Report on the Financial Outlook for Medicaid*, Centers for Medicare & Medicaid Services' Office of the Actuary, March 2012.

Medicaid Expenditures by Service Type

Figure 3 shows Medicaid expenditures by service type for FY2011. Long-term services and supports, which include nursing facility care and home- and community-based services, make up 24% of all Medicaid expenditures.[56] Managed care, which includes payments to managed care organizations,[57] primary care case management,[58] and non-comprehensive prepaid health plans,[59] also accounts for 24% of total Medicaid expenditures. Hospitals receive 13% of total Medicaid expenditures in return for services provided to Medicaid fee-for-service[60] enrollees at the payment rates set by states.[61]

Figure 3. Total Medicaid Expenditures by Service Type

FY2011

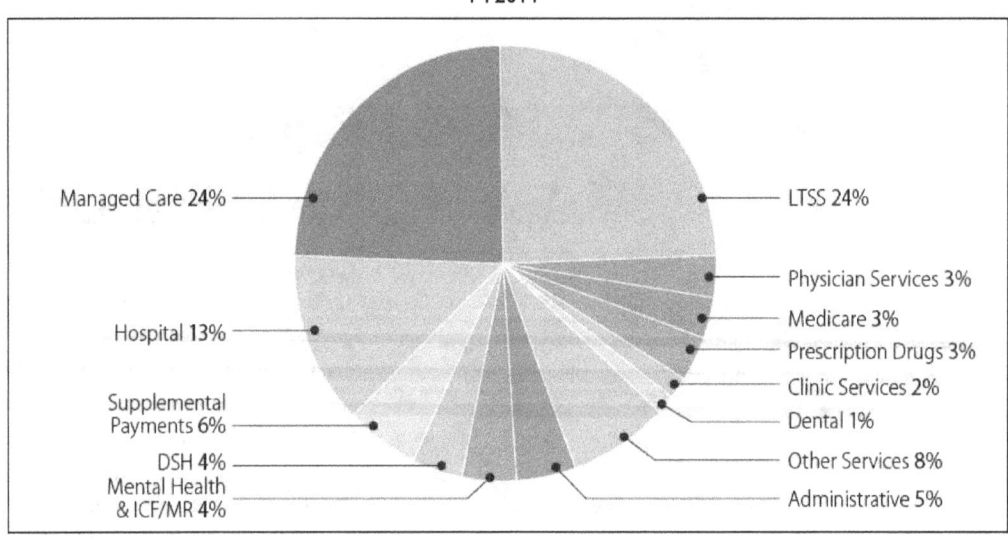

Source: Centers for Medicare & Medicaid Services, Form CMS-64 Data. Preliminary data as of April 16, 2012.

Note: Prescription drug expenditures are net rebates. "Other services" include any expenditure type that amounts to less than 1% of total Medicaid expenditures, such as laboratory services, rural health, targeted case

---

[56] For more information about long-term services and supports, see CRS Report R42345, *Long-Term Services and Supports Overview and Financing*, coordinated by Kirsten J. Colello.

[57] States contract with managed care organizations to provide a comprehensive package of benefits to enrolled Medicaid beneficiaries, primarily on a capitated basis (i.e., a set amount per enrollee regardless of the services utilized).

[58] Under primary care case management, states contract with primary care physicians to provide case management services to Medicaid enrollees. For these enrollees, other services are generally provided on a fee-for-service basis.

[59] States contract with health plans to provide non-comprehensive benefits (e.g., inpatient behavioral health care or dental care).

[60] There are two major types of service payment systems under Medicaid—fee-for-service (FFS) and managed care. The FFS system was the predominant system of care both within and outside of Medicaid until about the mid-1990s. Under FFS, beneficiaries have unrestricted provider choice; that is, they can seek services from any Medicaid participating provider. Hence, beneficiaries are largely responsible for their own medical care management and coordination. Under managed care, states purchase or establish a network of providers for their Medicaid enrollees through contracts with health plans and/or providers who agree to accept Medicaid patients and to meet certain requirements to ensure timely access to care.

[61] Hospitals also receive a significant portion of both the Medicaid DSH funding and the supplemental payments.

management, physical therapy, etc. LTSS comprise spending for nursing facility services, home health services, home- and community-based services, personal care services, etc. ICF/MR is an optional Medicaid benefit that enables states to provide comprehensive and individualized health care and rehabilitation services to individuals to promote their functional status and independence. Supplemental payments are Medicaid payments made to providers that are separate from and in addition to the standard payment rates for services rendered to Medicaid enrollees.

DSH: Disproportionate Share Hospital

ICF/MR: Intermediate Care Facility for individuals with Mental Retardation

LTSS: Long-Term Services and Supports

Factors Affecting Medicaid Expenditures

Medicaid expenditures are influenced by economic, demographic, and programmatic factors. Economic factors include health care prices, unemployment rates, and individuals' wages. Demographic factors include population growth and the age distribution of the population. Programmatic factors include state decisions regarding optional eligibility groups, optional services, and provider payment rates. Other factors include the number of eligible individuals who enroll, utilization of covered services, and enrollment in other health insurance programs (including Medicare and private health insurance). [62]

The Economy

Medicaid enrollment is affected by economic factors, which in turn have an impact on Medicaid expenditures. Medicaid is referred to as a countercyclical program, which means Medicaid enrollment growth tends to accelerate when the economy weakens and to slow when the economy gains strength. Researchers have estimated that for every 1% increase in the national unemployment rate, Medicaid enrollment increases by 1 million individuals. [63] People become eligible for Medicaid during economic downturns because they lose their job, have less income, or lose health benefits. [64]

Medicaid Enrollment

Since the beginning of the 2007-2009 recession, growth in Medicaid expenditures has been largely due to enrollment growth resulting from the higher unemployment rate. [65] The Bureau of

---

[62] Christopher J. Truffer, John D. Klemm, and Christian J. Wolfe, et al., *2011 Actuarial Report on the Financial Outlook for Medicaid*, Centers for Medicare & Medicaid Services' Office of the Actuary, March 2012; Andy Schneider and David Rousseau, *The Medicaid Resource Book*, The Kaiser Commission on Medicaid and the Uninsured, Publication Number 2236, January 17, 2003.

[63] John Holahan and A. Bowen Garrett, *Rising Unemployment, Medicaid and the Uninsured*, Kaiser Commission on Medicaid and the Uninsured, Publication #7850, January 2009.

[64] Rachel Garfield, Lisa Clemans-Cope, and Emily Lawton, et al., *Enrollment-Driven Expenditure Growth Medicaid Spending during the Economic Downturn, FFY2007-2010*, Kaiser Commission on Medicaid and the Uninsured, Publication #8309, May 2012.

[65] John Holahan, Lisa Clemans-Cope, and Emily Lawton, et al., *Medicaid Spending Growth of the Last Decade and the Great Recession, 2000-2009*, Kaiser Commission on Medicaid and the Uninsured, Publication 8152, February 2011; Rachel Garfield, Lisa Clemans-Cope, and Emily Lawton, et al., *Enrollment-Driven Expenditure Growth Medicaid Spending during the Economic Downturn, FFY2007-2010*, Kaiser Commission on Medicaid and the Uninsured, Publication #8309, May 2012.

Labor Statistics reported the seasonally adjusted national unemployment rate rose from 5.0% in December of 2007 to 9.5% in June of 2009, peaking at 10.0% in October 2010 (four months after the official end of the national recession).[66] Over roughly the same period, the estimated number of individuals ever enrolled[67] in Medicaid increased by 8.7%, from 58.8 million in FY2008 to an estimated 67.7 million in FY2010.[68] Medicaid enrollment growth occurred predominantly in the children and adult populations, while the Medicaid aged and disabled populations stayed relatively flat.[69]

Even though the recession officially ended in June 2009 and the economic environment has been improving, the unemployment rate remains high, which continues to affect Medicaid enrollment and expenditures. Total Medicaid expenditures increased by 5.9% in FY2008, 7.6% in FY2009, 6.0% in FY2010, and 6.5% in FY2011.[70]

Temporary FMAP Increase

As shown in **Figure 1**, the federal government covered the increase in total Medicaid expenditures from FY2009 through FY2011 through the temporary FMAP increase.[71] Federal Medicaid funding to states increased by $98.7 billion due to the temporary FMAP increase that was in place from October 1, 2008 through June 30, 2011. The temporary FMAP increase to states caused a shift in the federal and state shares of Medicaid expenditures, with the federal share of total Medicaid expenditures increasing from the typical 57% in FY2008 to 66% in FY2009, 67% in FY2010, and an estimated 63% in FY2011.[72]

The temporary FMAP increase also caused shifts in the annual percent change in the federal and state Medicaid expenditures (**Figure 4**).

---

[66] Bureau of Labor Statistics, *Labor Force Statistics from the Current Population* Survey, available at http://data.bls.gov/pdq/SurveyOutputServlet?data_tool=latest_numbers&series_id=LNS14000000.

[67] Since there is a lot of turnover in the Medicaid program, Medicaid enrollment measured in different ways can produce vastly different enrollment figures. Medicaid enrollment could be measured by "ever enrolled" persons (i.e., the number of people covered by Medicaid for any period of time during the year), "person-year equivalents" (i.e., the average enrollment over the course of the year), and "point-in-time" (i.e., the number of Medicaid enrollees at a specified date). The annual count of Medicaid enrollees measured by "ever enrolled" persons will always exceed Medicaid enrollment measured by "person-year equivalents."

[68] MACPAC, *March 2011 Report to the Congress on Medicaid and CHIP*, Table 2, March 2011. Federal fiscal year 2008 ran from October 1, 2007, through September 30, 2008, and federal fiscal year 2010 ran from October 1, 2009, through September 30, 2010.

[69] John Holahan, Lisa Clemans-Cope, and Emily Lawton, et al., *Medicaid Spending Growth of the Last Decade and the Great Recession, 2000-2009*, Kaiser Commission on Medicaid and the Uninsured, Publication 8152, February 2011.

[70] CRS calculation based on Form CMS-64 data from the Centers for Medicare & Medicaid. The FY2011 CMS-64 data is not finalized, and the data used is as of April 16, 2012. Not all of these increases are attributed to the economic environment.

[71] The temporary FMAP increase was originally provided through the American Recovery and Reinvestment Act of 2009 (ARRA, P.L. 111-5) for nine fiscal quarters (October 1, 2008 through December 31, 2010), and the temporary FMAP increase was extended by six months (January 1, 2011 through June 30, 2011) at a phased down level through P.L. 111-226. For more information about the temporary FMAP increase, see CRS Report RL32950, *Medicaid The Federal Medical Assistance Percentage (FMAP)*, by Alison Mitchell and Evelyne P. Baumrucker.

[72] CRS calculations based on Form CMS-64 data from the Centers for Medicare & Medicaid. The FY2011 CMS-64 data is not finalized, and the data used is as of April 16, 2012.

Figure 4. Annual Percent Change in Federal and State Medicaid Expenditures

FY1998 to FY2012 Estimate

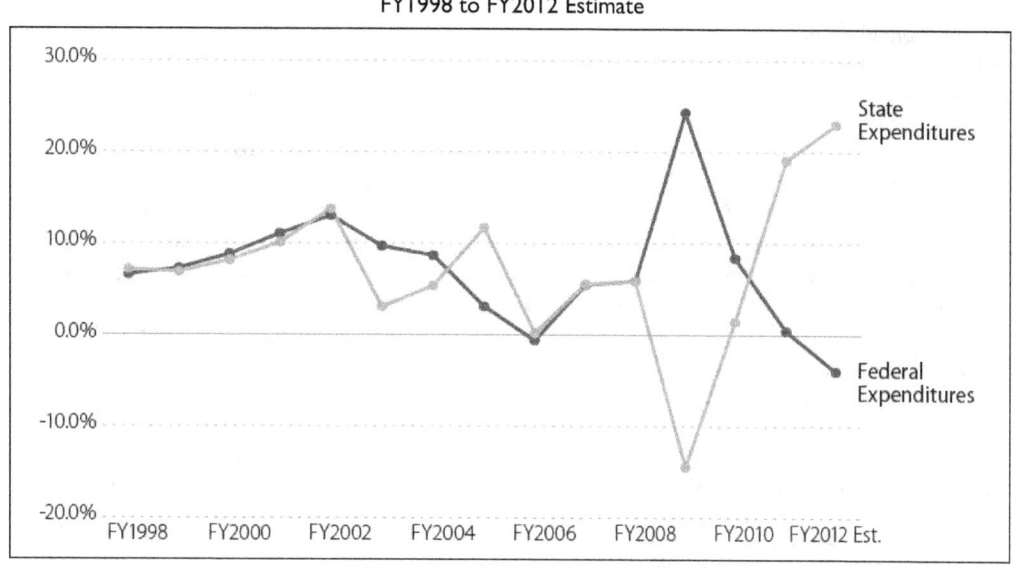

Source: Centers for Medicare & Medicaid Services, Form CMS-64 Data. The Form CMS-64 data for FY2011 is not fina ized, and the data used is as of April 16, 2012 (FY1997 to FY2011). Christopher J. Truffer, John D. Klemm, and Christian J. Wolfe, et al., *2011 Actuarial Report on the Financial Outlook for Medicaid*, Centers for Medicare & Medicaid Services' Office of the Actuary, March 2012 (FY2012 estimate).

Prior to the 2001 recession, when additional federal funding was provided, federal and state Medicaid expenditures grew at the same rate. When additional federal funds were provided in FY2003 and FY2004, federal funds increased more than state funds. When the recession-related federal funds expired in FY2005, state expenditures increased more than federal Medicaid expenditures. In FY2006 through FY2008, federal and state Medicaid expenditures returned to increasing at the same rate. The temporary FMAP increase began October 1, 2008 causing federal Medicaid expenditures to increase significantly in FY2009 and FY2010 (24% and 8%, respectively), while state Medicaid expenditures decreased by 14% in FY2009 and were flat in FY2010.[73] The temporary increase phased down beginning January 1, 2011 and expired June 30, 2011 (three-quarters of the way through FY2011), which caused state Medicaid expenditures to increase 19% in FY2011 while federal expenditures were relatively flat.[74] In FY2012, state Medicaid expenditures are projected to increase 23% and federal Medicaid expenditures are estimated to decrease by 4%.[75]

The shifts in the annual percent changes for federal and state Medicaid expenditures were more dramatic during the most recent recession because the federal government provided significantly more fiscal relief to states relative to the fiscal relief provided for the 2001 recession.

---

[73] CRS calculation based on Form CMS-64 data from the Centers for Medicare & Medicaid. The FY2011 CMS-64 data is not finalized, and the data used is as of April 16, 2012.

[74] CRS calculation based on Form CMS-64 data from the Centers for Medicare & Medicaid. The FY2011 CMS-64 data is not finalized, and the data used is as of April 16, 2012.

[75] Christopher J. Truffer, John D. Klemm, and Christian J. Wolfe, et al., *2011 Actuarial Report on the Financial Outlook for Medicaid*, Centers for Medicare & Medicaid Services' Office of the Actuary, March 2012.

State Variability in Medicaid Spending

There is considerable variation in Medicaid spending from state to state. Some of the state variation is caused by demographic differences, such as state population and proportion of low-income residents. However, state variation in Medicaid per-enrollee expenditures is significant.

In order to participate in Medicaid, the federal government requires states to cover certain mandatory populations and benefits, but allows states to cover optional populations and services. In fact, an analysis of FY2001 Medicaid expenditures found that 61% of Medicaid expenditures are optional. Specifically, the analysis found that 39% of Medicaid expenditures were mandatory services for mandatory populations, while the remaining 61% of Medicaid expenditures were either optional services for mandatory groups (18%), mandatory services for optional groups (30%), or optional services for optional groups (12%).[76] Some of the sickest and poorest Medicaid enrollees are considered "optional," and many "optional benefits" provided under Medicaid often are integral health care services.[77]

State policy choices regarding optional populations and optional services cause variation in Medicaid spending. However, there are other reasons Medicaid spending varies from state to state.

Some of the state variation in Medicaid per-enrollee expenditures is due to differences across states in the demographics of Medicaid enrollees. For instance, states with lower-than-average proportions of elderly and disabled Medicaid enrollees and higher-than-average proportions of Medicaid enrollees that are low-income children and adults would be expected to have lower than average per-enrollee Medicaid expenditures.[78]

State variation in Medicaid per-enrollee expenditures is also due to variation in utilization and provider payment rates.[79] One analysis of disabled Medicaid enrollees found that utilization accounted for a significant amount of the variation in per-enrollee Medicaid expenditures. Specifically, the variation was attributed to utilization of inpatient hospital services and prescription drugs. The study found little difference in the per-enrollee Medicaid expenditures for ambulatory visits, such as physician, outpatient hospital, and clinic services.[80]

---

[76] Does not add to 61% due to rounding.

[77] Numbers may not exactly sum to totals, due to rounding. Anna Sommers, Arunabh Ghosh, and David Rousseau, *Medicaid Enrollment and Spending by "Mandatory" and "Optional" Eligibility and Benefit Categories*, Kaiser Commission on Medicaid and the Uninsured, June 2005.

[78] Todd P. Gilmer and Richard G. Kronick, "Differences in the Volume of Services and in Prices Drive Big Variation in Medicaid Spending Among U.S. States and Regions," *Health Affairs*, vol. 30, no. 7 (July 2011).

[79] Todd P. Gilmer and Richard G. Kronick, "Differences in the Volume of Services and in Prices Drive Big Variation in Medicaid Spending Among U.S. States and Regions," *Health Affairs*, vol. 30, no. 7 (July 2011).

[80] To maximize the comparability of the sample across states, the study population was Medicaid-only disabled Medicaid enrollees on cash assistance that received Medicaid services on a fee-for-service basis. Todd P. Gilmer and Richard G. Kronick, "Differences in the Volume of Services and in Prices Drive Big Variation in Medicaid Spending Among U.S. States and Regions," *Health Affairs*, vol. 30, no. 7 (July 2011).

Projected Medicaid Expenditures

Over the next ten years, Medicaid expenditures had been projected to increase significantly, mainly due to the changes enacted by the Patient Protection and Affordable Care Act (ACA, P.L. 111-148 as amended) with the Medicaid provisions in ACA representing the most considerable federal legislative change to Medicaid since its enactment in 1965.[81] However, on June 28, 2012, the United States Supreme Court issued its decision in *National Federation of Independent Business v. Sebelius*, which is expected to reduce the original estimated cost of the ACA Medicaid expansion.

ACA Medicaid Expansion

The most noteworthy ACA change to Medicaid is the expansion of Medicaid eligibility to adults under age 65 with income up to 133% of the federal poverty level (FPL) (effectively 138% FPL with the Modified Adjusted Gross Income 5% FPL income disregard).[82] Originally, the assumption was that all states would implement the ACA Medicaid expansion in 2014 as required in statute because implementing the ACA Medicaid expansion was required in order for states to receive *any* federal Medicaid funding. However, on June 28, 2012, the United States Supreme Court issued its decision in *National Federation of Independent Business v. Sebelius*, finding that the federal government cannot terminate the federal Medicaid funding states are receiving for their current Medicaid program if a state refuses to implement the ACA Medicaid expansion. If a state accepts the new ACA Medicaid expansion funds, it must abide by the new expansion coverage rules, but, based on the Court's opinion, it appears that a state can refuse to participate in the expansion without losing any of its current federal Medicaid matching funds.

Since the Supreme Court ruling, some states have stated their intention to implement the ACA Medicaid expansion, other states have asserted that they will not implement the expansion, and most states remain uncommitted.

Prior to the Supreme Court decision, when it was assumed all states would implement the ACA Medicaid expansion, the Congressional Budget Office (CBO) and the Joint Committee on Taxation (JCT) estimated that the ACA Medicaid expansion would increase Medicaid and the State Children's Health Insurance Program (CHIP) enrollment by 13 million in FY2014 increasing to 17 million by FY2022, which CBO estimated would increase federal Medicaid expenditures by $931 billion from FY2012 to FY2022.[83]

On July 24, 2012, CBO and JCT updated their estimates for the ACA Medicaid expansion taking into consideration the Supreme Court ruling.[84] According to the updated estimate, in each year

---

[81] Christopher J. Truffer, John D. Klemm, and Christian J. Wolfe, et al., *2011 Actuarial Report on the Financial Outlook for Medicaid*, Centers for Medicare & Medicaid Services' Office of the Actuary, March 2012.

[82] Historically, Medicaid eligibility was generally limited to low-income children, pregnant women, parents of dependent children, the elderly, and people with disabilities. For more information about the ACA changes to Medicaid, see CRS Report R41210, *Medicaid and the State Children's Health Insurance Program (CHIP) Provisions in ACA Summary and Timeline*, by Evelyne P. Baumrucker et al.

[83] Figure reflects average annual enrollment. Congressional Budget Office, *Updated Estimates for the Insurance Coverage Provisions of the Affordable Care Act*, March 2012.

[84] The CBO and JCT estimate does not make state-by-state predictions regarding which states will implement the ACA Medicaid expansion or not.

---

between FY2014 and FY2022, the number of individuals covered by the ACA Medicaid expansion will be 5 to 7 million less than estimated before the Supreme Court decision.[85] Specifically, CBO estimates the ACA Medicaid expansion will increase Medicaid and CHIP enrollment by 7 million in FY2014 increasing to 11 million by FY2022.[86]

As shown in **Figure 5**, from FY2014 to FY2022, federal Medicaid expenditures resulting from the ACA Medicaid expansion are estimated to be $642 billion, which is $288 billion less than the cost estimated prior to the Supreme Court's decision. States' spending due to the ACA Medicaid expansion is estimated to be $41 billion from FY2012 to FY2022, which is $32 billion less than the amount estimated prior to the Supreme Court decision.[87]

Figure 5. Estimated Federal Medicaid and CHIP Outlays for the ACA Medicaid Expansion Before and After the Supreme Court Decision

FY2014 to FY2022

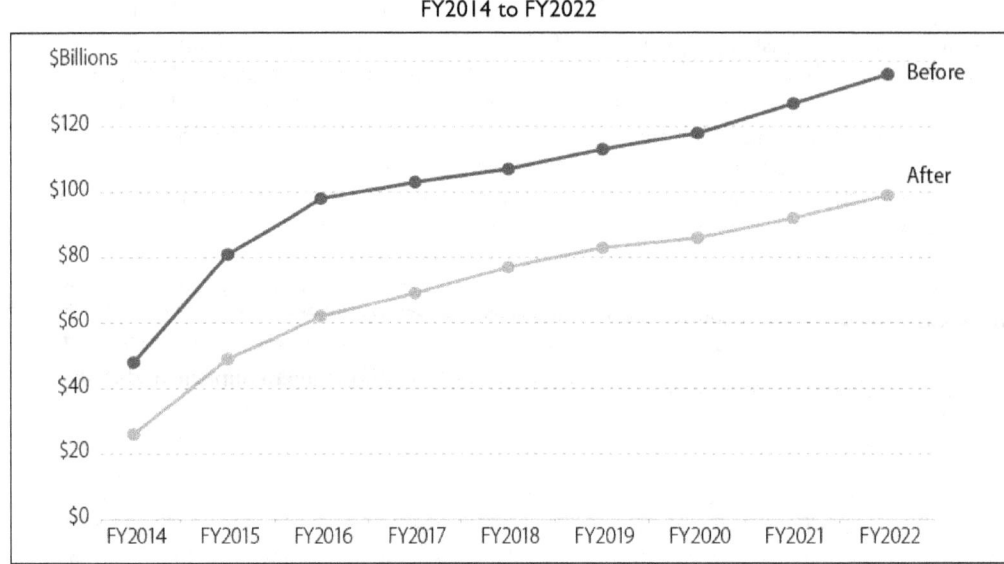

Note: Figure represents outlays in Medicaid only. CBO and JCT estimates that lower projected Medicaid spending due to some states not implementing the ACA Medicaid expansion would be offset by increased spending for the ACA insurance coverage provisions.

Source: Congressional Budget Office, *Estimates for the Insurance Coverage Provisions of the Affordable Care Act Updated for the Recent Supreme Court Decision,* July 2012; Congressional Budget Office, *Updated Estimates for the Insurance Coverage Provisions of the Affordable Care Act,* March 2012.

---

[85] The difference in the estimated number of individuals covered by the ACA Medicaid expansion before and after the Supreme Court decision varies in each year between FY2014 to FY2022. The following is the difference between the two estimates in each year: FY2014 = 6 million, FY2015 = 6 million, FY2016 = 7 million, FY2017 = 6 million, FY2018 = 5 million, FY2019 = 5 million, FY2020 = 6 million, FY2021 = 6 million, and FY2022 = 6 million.

[86] Congressional Budget Office, *Estimates for the Insurance Coverage Provisions of the Affordable Care Act Updated for the Recent Supreme Court Decision,* July 2012.

[87] Ibid.

Other ACA Provisions

ACA makes a number of other changes to the Medicaid program that are expected to impact Medicaid expenditures.[88] Some ACA provisions that are expected to increase Medicaid expenditures include payments to the territories, the new Community First Choice Option,[89] the removal of barriers to providing home- and community-based services, and the extension of the Money Follows the Person demonstration.[90] Other provisions in ACA are expected to reduce Medicaid expenditures, including changes to prescription drug coverage and DSH payments.[91]

Current Issues

House Budget Resolution Proposed Block Grant

On March 20, 2012, Representative Paul Ryan, the Chairman of the House Budget Committee, released the Chairman's mark of the FY2013 House budget resolution.[92] Additional detail on budgetary objectives and justifications was provided in Chairman Ryan's report entitled, "The Path to Prosperity: A Blueprint for American Renewal," issued the same day.[93] The House Budget Committee considered the Chairman's mark on March 21, 2012, and voted 19-18 to report the budget resolution to the full House.[94] H.Con.Res. 112 was introduced in the House March 23, 2012, and was accompanied by the House Budget Committee report (H.Rept. 112-421). The House agreed to H.Con.Res. 112 on March 29, 2012, by a vote of 228 to 191.

The committee report includes illustrative examples for achieving budget savings, such as a change in the structure of the Medicare and Medicaid programs and the repeal of many of the provisions in ACA.[95] One of the proposals would restructure the Medicaid program from an individual entitlement[96] to a block grant.[97] According to CBO's long-term analysis of the block

---

[88] For more information about the other ACA provisions impacting the Medicaid program, see CRS Report R41210, *Medicaid and the State Children's Health Insurance Program (CHIP) Provisions in ACA Summary and Timeline*, by Evelyne P. Baumrucker et al.

[89] Community First Choice Option is a state plan option in which states can offer consumer-directed personal care attendant services and receive an increased federal match rate of 6 percentage points for doing so.

[90] The Money Follows the Person demonstration helps states rebalance their long-term care systems by transitioning people with Medicaid from institutions to the community.

[91] Congressional Budget Office, *Selected CBO Publications Related to Health Care Legislation, 2009-2010*, December 22, 2010.

[92] The Chairman's mark may be found at http://budget.house.gov/UploadedFiles/chairmans_mark_FY013.pdf.

[93] This report may be found at http://budget.house.gov/UploadedFiles/Pathtoprosperity2013.pdf.

[94] The Concurrent Resolution on the Budget as Recorded was made available on March 22, 2012, http://budget.house.gov/UploadedFiles/Concurrent_Resolution_Budget_FY_2013.pdf.

[95] For more information on these proposals, see CRS Report R42441, *Overview of Health Care Changes in the FY2013 Budget Proposal Offered by House Budget Committee Chairman Ryan*, by Patricia A. Davis, Alison Mitchell, and Bernadette Fernandez.

[96] Individual entitlement means that individuals who meet state eligibility requirements, which must also meet federal minimum requirements, are entitled to Medicaid.

[97] Historically, the term block grant has been used to mean programs for which the federal government provides state governments with a fixed amount of federal funds generally for administering and providing certain services to targeted groups of individuals.

---

grant proposal, when compared with long-term estimates of current law, combined federal spending for Medicaid, CHIP, and the exchange subsidies would be 76% to 78% lower in FY2050.[98] Since spending on CHIP and exchange subsidies is expected to be small relative to federal spending on Medicaid over this time period, most of the reduction will come from the Medicaid program.[99]

Proponents of the block grant model suggest that this design would make federal Medicaid spending more predictable and provide states with stronger incentives to control the cost of their Medicaid programs. Additionally, this design could relieve some of the cost burden to states by removing certain federal Medicaid requirements.[100]

According to CBO, the implications of converting Medicaid to a block grant program would depend on how states respond to the change. With the added flexibility provided under Chairman Ryan's proposal, states could improve the efficiency of their Medicaid programs. However, even with significant efficiency gains, the magnitude of the federal Medicaid spending reductions under this proposal would make it difficult for states to maintain their current Medicaid programs.[101] As a result, states would have to weigh the impact of maintaining current Medicaid service levels against other state priorities for spending. States could choose to constrain Medicaid expenditures by reducing provider reimbursement rates, limiting benefit packages, or restricting eligibility. These types of programmatic changes could also affect access to and the quality of medical care for Medicaid enrollees.

Federal Deficit Reduction

In FY2012, federal Medicaid expenditures account for almost 8% of all federal spending.[102] As a result, controlling federal Medicaid spending has been a focus of federal deficit reduction proposals, such as the House Budget Resolution (discussed above in "House Budget Resolution Proposed Block Grant") and the National Commission on Fiscal Reform.

The National Commission on Fiscal Reform final report included savings from Medicaid totaling $58 billion over 10 years. The savings came from eliminating states' ability to fund Medicaid through provider taxes, covering dual-eligibles under managed care arrangements, and giving states additional fiscal responsibility for administrative costs.[103]

---

[98] Congressional Budget Office, The Long-Term Budgetary Impact of Paths for Federal Revenues and Spending Specified by Chairman Ryan, March 2012.

[99] According to CBO estimates of mandatory outlays in FY2022, the combined federal outlays for Medicaid, health insurance subsidies, exchanges, and related spending, and CHIP would total to $715 billion, and federal Medicaid expenditures would comprise 85% of that total amount. Congressional Budget Office, *The Budget and Economic Outlook FY2012 to FY2022*, January 2012.

[100] For additional information on block grants, see CRS Report R40486, *Block Grants Perspectives and Controversies*, by Robert Jay Dilger and Eugene Boyd.

[101] Congressional Budget Office, The Long-Term Budgetary Impact of Paths for Federal Revenues and Spending Specified by Chairman Ryan, March 2012.

[102] Office of Management and Budget, *Historical Tables Budget of the U.S. Government, Fiscal Year 2012*.

[103] National Commission on Fiscal Reform, *The Moment of Truth Report of the National Commission on Fiscal Responsibility and Reform*, December 1, 2010, http://www.fiscalcommission.gov/sites/fiscalcommission.gov/files/documents/TheMomentofTruth12_1_2010.pdf.

Additionally, in February 2012, the President's FY2013 budget was released, which included a number of Medicaid provisions estimated by the Administration to reduce federal Medicaid expenditures by $55.7 billion over the next 10 years.[104] The Medicaid provisions include limiting states' ability to utilize provider taxes[105] in financing the state share of Medicaid expenditures; replacing the current federal Medicaid financing structure with a blended FMAP rate;[106] limiting Medicaid reimbursement of durable medical equipment; re-basing Medicaid DSH payments; expanding state flexibility to provide benchmark benefit packages; extending transitional medical assistance; and establishing hold harmless for federal poverty guidelines. In addition, the President's FY2013 budget includes a number of program integrity proposals that are estimated to reduce federal Medicaid expenditures by $3.2 billion from FY2013 through FY2022.[107]

To the extent that federal Medicaid expenditures are reduced, in most cases states would need to increase their share of Medicaid to maintain their current Medicaid programs. This will be difficult for states that are already struggling to fund their current share of Medicaid expenditures, due to the adverse impacts of the recession on state budgets. Faced with this situation, states would have to weigh the impact of maintaining current Medicaid service levels against other state spending priorities.

State Fiscal Conditions

During periods of economic downturn, state Medicaid programs face dual pressures. First, program enrollment increases at a faster rate when job and income losses lead more people to become eligible for Medicaid. Second, it can be more difficult to finance the state share of Medicaid costs because state revenue growth generally weakens during economic downturns.

When viewed nationally, Medicaid is the largest or second-largest item in state budgets depending on how it is measured. In terms of *total* state spending (i.e., funds from all state and federal sources), in SFY 2011, Medicaid was the largest component of the budget at an estimated 23.6% of *total* state spending. However, Medicaid is the second-largest component in terms of state *general fund* spending (i.e., the portion that states must finance on their own through taxes and other means). In SFY2011, Medicaid expenditures were an estimated 17.4% of state general fund spending, while elementary and secondary education spending was 35.0%.[108]

Throughout the recession, Medicaid expenditures grew as a percent of total state spending and shrank as a percent of state general fund spending because the federal government absorbed most of the recession-related increase in Medicaid expenditures through the temporary increase to

---

[104] Department of Health and Human Services, *Fiscal Year 2013 Budget in Brief Strengthening Health and Opportunity for All Americans*, February 2012.

[105] For more information about Medicaid provider taxes, see CRS Report RS22843, *Medicaid Provider Taxes*, by Alison Mitchell.

[106] Details regarding the proposed blended FMAP rate are not available, but essentially the blended rate would replace the current patchwork of federal matching rates with a single federal matching rate for all Medicaid expenditures. Since the blended rate was proposed in the context of federal deficit actions, it is expected that the proposed blended rate would provide budgetary savings to the federal government.

[107] For more information about the President's FY2013 budget proposals impacting Medicaid, see CRS Report R42368, *Centers for Medicare & Medicaid Services President's FY2013 Budget*, coordinated by Alison Mitchell and Paulette C. Morgan.

[108] The SFY2011 data are based on 50-state preliminary actual survey data presented in the following report: National Governors Association and National Association of State Budget Officers, *The Fiscal Survey of States*, Fall 2011.

FMAP rates.[109] However, with the phase out of the temporary increase to FMAP rates in SFY2011, Medicaid expenditures as a share of state general fund spending grew from 15.8% in SFY2010 to an estimated 17.4% in SFY2011.[110]

While total Medicaid spending (i.e., including both federal and state spending) grew throughout the recession, total state tax revenues are estimated to have declined by 10.2% from the fourth quarter of 2007 to the fourth quarter of 2009.[111] Even with the temporary increase to FMAP rates moderating the impact of Medicaid expenditure growth on state general fund spending, many states faced budget deficits. A study from the Government Accountability Office notes that while these fiscal tensions existed for nearly all states during the economic downturn, any given state's capacity to finance the state share of Medicaid costs differed based on variables such as the state's economic condition, revenue structure, Medicaid program design, etc. Moreover, among states, economic downturns varied widely in their onset, depth, and duration, and generally do not coincide exactly with national recessions.[112]

Even though the national recession officially ended in June 2009, state tax revenues did not start increasing until the first fiscal quarter of 2010. States have experienced eight consecutive quarters of revenue growth, but total state revenues only surpassed peak levels from 2007 in the fourth quarter of 2011.[113] As a result, nearly every state implemented at least one new Medicaid cost containment policy in SFY2010, SFY2011, and SFY2012.[114] Because states are prohibited from curbing the cost of Medicaid by restricting eligibility standards due to the maintenance of effort (MOE) requirements initially enacted under ARRA and later expanded and extended under ACA,[115] over the past few years, states have focused cost containment strategies on reducing provider rates, making changes to their benefit packages, or implementing limitations on the use of benefits.[116]

---

[109] The American Recovery and Reinvestment Act of 2009 (ARRA, P.L. 111-5) included a temporary increase to FMAP rates to help states maintain their Medicaid programs and free up funds that states would have otherwise used for Medicaid to address other state budgetary needs. The temporary FMAP rate increase was originally provided for nine fiscal quarters (October 1, 2008 through December 31, 2010), and the temporary FMAP rate increase was extended by six months (January 1, 2011 through June 30, 2011) at a phased down level through P.L. 111-226. For more information about the temporary FMAP rate increase, see CRS Report RL32950, *Medicaid: The Federal Medical Assistance Percentage (FMAP)*, by Alison Mitchell and Evelyne P. Baumrucker.

[110] National Association of State Budget Officers, *Fiscal Year 2010 State Expenditure Report Examining Fiscal 2009-2011 State Spending*, December 2011; National Governors Association and National Association of State Budget Officers, *The Fiscal Survey of States*, Fall 2011.

[111] U.S. Government Accountability Office, *Medicaid Improving Responsiveness to Federal Assistance to States During Economic Downturns*, GAO-11-395, March 2011.

[112] U.S. Government Accountability Office, *Medicaid Improving Responsiveness to Federal Assistance to States During Economic Downturns*, GAO-11-395, March 2011.

[113] Lucy Dadayan, *Tax Revenues Surpass Previous Peak But Growth Softens Once Again*, The Nelson A. Rockefeller Institute of Government at the University of Albany, State Revenue Report No. 87, April 2012.

[114] Kaiser Commission on Medicaid and the Uninsured, *A Mid-Year State Medicaid Budget Update for FY 2012 and A Look Forward to FY2013*, February 2012; Vernon K. Smith, Kathleen Gifford, and Eileen Ellis, et al., *Moving Ahead Amid Fiscal Challenges A Look at Medicaid Spending, Coverage and Policy Trends, Results from a 50-State Medicaid Budget Survey for State Fiscal Years 2011 and 2012*, Kaiser Commission on Medicaid and the Uninsured, October 2011.

[115] For more information about the MOE requirements, see CRS Report R41835, *Medicaid and CHIP Maintenance of Effort (MOE) Requirements and Responses*, by Evelyne P. Baumrucker.

[116] Kaiser Commission on Medicaid and the Uninsured, *A Mid-Year State Medicaid Budget Update for FY 2012 and A Look Forward to FY2013*, February 2012; Vernon K. Smith, Kathleen Gifford, and Eileen Ellis, et al., *Moving Ahead Amid Fiscal Challenges A Look at Medicaid Spending, Coverage and Policy Trends, Results from a 50-State Medicaid* (continued...)

Due to Medicaid's federal/state financing structure, for states to generate $1 of savings in the state share of Medicaid spending, they would have to reduce their overall Medicaid spending by $2 to almost $4, depending on each state's regular FMAP rate. For example, in a state with a FMAP rate of 50%, to obtain state-share savings in the amount of $20 million the state would have to reduce total federal and state Medicaid spending by approximately $40 million. In a state with a FMAP rate of 65%, to obtain state-share savings in the amount of $20 million the state would have to reduce total federal and state share Medicaid spending by approximately $57 million. The degree to which a state is willing to cut the state share of its Medicaid spending might depend in part on the loss of federal dollars it would also face as a result of these reductions. This issue is a larger issue for states with higher FMAP rates, which have to cut their Medicaid program significantly to find small amounts of savings in state share.[117]

Historically, it has taken three to five years from the onset of a recession for state revenues to recover, and there is evidence that states' recovery from the most recent recession will take longer than other recent recessions.[118] It is currently three years after the recession officially ended, and states are reporting budget gaps for at least the next two years (SFY2013 and SFY2014).[119]

The projected budget gaps only convey part of the fiscal challenges for states because the reported gaps do not reflect the underfunding of pensions and retiree health care liabilities. Also, in recent years, budget gaps have sometimes been reduced temporarily by nonrecurring resources, such as rainy day funds.[120]

Prior to the recession, Medicaid was a fiscal challenge for states because Medicaid spending was growing faster than state revenues. This problem continued through the recession, and the trend is expected to continue for the foreseeable future.[121]

The Centers for Medicare & Medicaid Services' Office of the Actuary recently estimated Medicaid expenditures would increase by an average annual amount of 8.1% from FY2011 to FY2020 if the ACA Medicaid expansion were fully implemented by all states and 6.6% over the same period if costs attributable to ACA are excluded.[122] Even at the 6.6% growth rate, Medicaid expenditure growth would significantly outpace historic growth rates for state revenues.[123] Thus,

---

(...continued)

Budget Survey for State Fiscal Years 2011 and 2012, Kaiser Commission on Medicaid and the Uninsured, October 2011.

[117] Kaiser Commission on Medicaid and the Uninsured, *State Medicaid Agencies Prepare for Health Care Reform While Continuing to Face Challenges from the Recession.* August 2010.

[118] Donald J. Boyd, *The State of State Budgets*, The Nelson A. Rockefeller Institute of Government, National Conference of State Legislatures Fiscal Leaders Seminar, San Diego, CA, December 9, 2009.

[119] "Although not all state budget offices have completed forecasts, thus far 19 states are projecting $30.7 billion in budget gaps for fiscal 2013 and 11 states are projecting $23.2 billion in budget gaps for fiscal 2014." National Governors Association and National Association of State Budget Officers, *The Fiscal Survey of States*, Spring 2012.

[120] Budget stabilization or "rainy day" funds allow states to set aside excess revenue for use in times of unexpected revenue shortfall or budget deficit. State Budget Crisis Task Force, *Report of the State Budget Crisis Task Force*, July 2012.

[121] U.S. Government Accountability Office, *State and Local Governments' Fiscal Outlook April 2012 Update*, GAO-12-523SP, April 2012. State Budget Crisis Task Force, *Report of the State Budget Crisis Task Force*, July 2012.

[122] Christopher J. Truffer, John D. Klemm, and Christian J. Wolfe, et al., *2011 Actuarial Report on the Financial Outlook for Medicaid*, Centers for Medicare & Medicaid Services' Office of the Actuary, March 2012.

[123] State Budget Crisis Task Force, *Report of the State Budget Crisis Task Force*, July 2012.

---

while the fiscal environment for states is improving, states continue to face challenges with the ongoing costs of Medicaid and the potential future costs of the ACA Medicaid expansion.

Author Contact Information

Alison Mitchell
Analyst in Health Care Financing
amitchell@crs.loc.gov, 7-0152